JULIANNE ROSS

LIVING WITH YOUR BODY

**The Ultimate Guide on How to Have
a Healthy and Beautiful Body Through
Eating the Right Foods and Exercise**

Descrierea CIP a Bibliotecii Naţionale a României
JULIANNE ROSS
    **LIVING WITH YOUR BODY. The Ultimate Guide on How
to Have a Healthy and Beautiful Body Through Eating the
Right Foods and Exercise** / Julianne Ross – Bucharest: Editura
My Ebook, 2021
    ISBN

JULIANNE ROSS

LIVING WITH YOUR BODY
**The Ultimate Guide on How to Have
a Healthy and Beautiful Body Through
Eating the Right Foods and Exercise**

My Ebook Publishing House
Bucharest, 2021

TABLE OF CONTENTS

INTRODUCTION

It is not a question anymore of why is it necessary to have a strong and healthy body, it is a question of how we are going to sustain a healthy body. Generally, we know the benefits of having a healthy body, however many of us don't know how to sustain a healthy body. This is actually the true challenge, and once you are able to master the concept of keeping your body fit, you'll be able to fight any physical, mental and emotional disability better than the others.

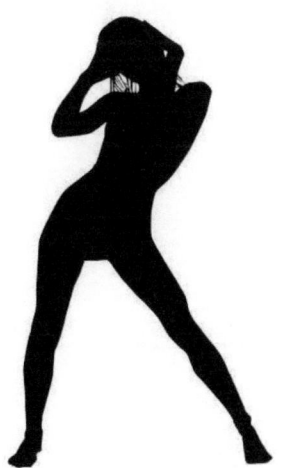

CHAPTER 1

INTRODUCTION

Synopsis

So how do we sustain a healthy body? Generally, we can keep our body in good shape when we feed it with the right nutrition and at the same time we do regular exercise. Physical exercise is known to be very effective in keeping our body working properly. This is because a good exercise can strengthen the immune system which is responsible in defending our body against any diseases. Furthermore, it can also improve our body's digestion, blood circulation and musculoskeletal function.

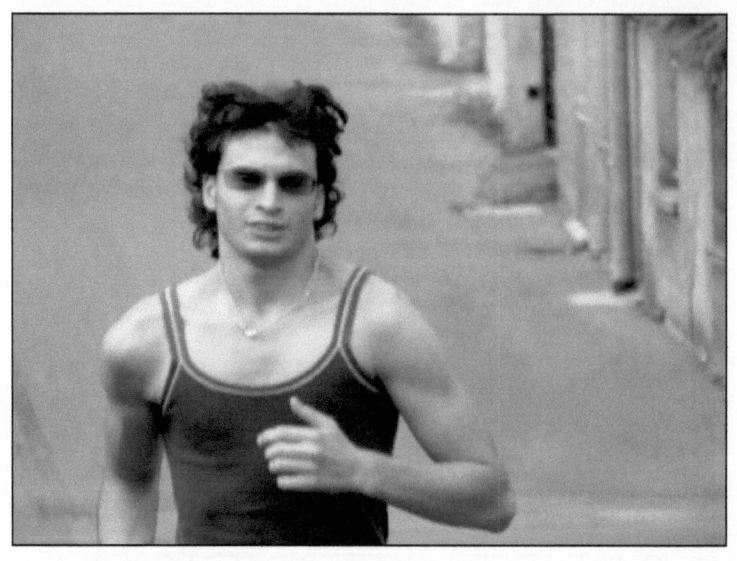

The Basics

Another way of keeping our body healthy is to allow it to have full rest. Through the night, our body is working to repair and maintain body parts that are not functioning well. Therefore, depriving ourselves of sleep will cause us to feel weak and eventually feel fatigued. On the other hand, when we are fully rested our body can easily repair cells and gain enough strength for the next day.

Furthermore, when our body is consistently healthy we can handle stress easily and we will become more resilient to any infection. In addition, a well maintained body can effectively fight back chronic diseases such as high blood pressure, heart disease, diabetes, cancer and many more. More than that, these diseases can be prevented when we are maintaining healthy body through exercise and proper nutrition.

On the other hand, staying fit also means keeping a good body build. The more time we spend exercising the more calories we burn. Based on studies, when we exercise for at least 30 minutes daily, our food intake will be reduced from high to average. This also means that our calorie intake will be balanced, which in result will give us a healthy and controlled weight.

CHAPTER 2

MAINTAINING A HEALTHY WEIGHT WITH THE RIGHT FOODS AND NOT DIETING

Synopsis

When it comes to the subject of weight loss, the first thing that comes out in our minds is dieting. However, there are arguments that came out that it is not actually dieting that will help us maintain a healthy weight but it is eating the right foods. Common sense would tell us that when we eat less nutritional food, we are not feeding our body with enough nutrients that it needs to function properly. Therefore, when our body is not properly nourished, there is a tendency that we get sick because our body parts cannot function well.

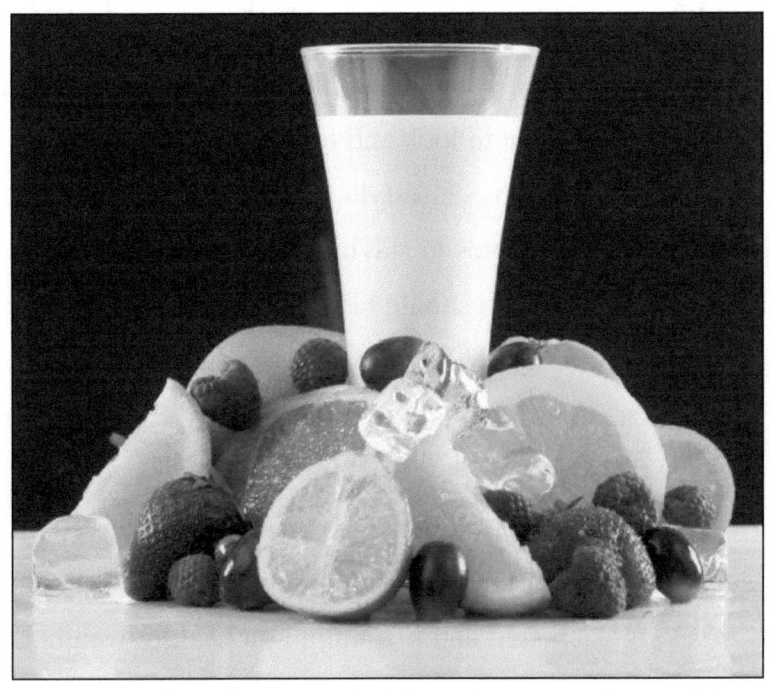

Eat Healthy

Again, the answer to weight problems is not short term dietary programs that give out fast results, instead the key is feeding our body with the right food, having healthy lifestyles and engaging ourselves in regular physical exercise. In short, we don't need to get quick results, we need to get lasting results through the natural way.

The good thing about losing weight the right way is that it does not only give us long-lasting effects, it will also help us to stay healthy and look younger as we age. Here's how to get started with eating right to look and feel right.

Choose a healthy lifestyle over a short-term diet. Apparently, when it comes to staying fit and healthy there is no such thing as quick fix. It should be done gradually and properly to get permanent results. Although, prevalent diets can help you get a good start in your weight loss objective, it's definitely not the package that will give you enduring benefits.

Establish a support group who will help inspire, remind and support you with your plans. You can combine people and tools in taking each step and maintaining a healthy weight. Ask any of your friends or family members to be your support group and let your plan be known to them so that they can guide you all throughout. Also, to complete your support system you may want to add a weight loss tool that can help you trace your calorie intake and more.

Make a good change slowly but constantly. Remember, it is not about the thing that you do that will make you successful in maintaining your health but it is how persistent you are in doing it. Therefore, it is also important that you make achievable and effective goals in order for you stay motivated. When

14

temptation attacks, focus more on the long term benefits that you will receive rather than the temporary ones.

Lastly, consider experimenting in order for you to discover the right diet that can supply your needs aside from keeping you in great shape. This is because whatever you do, finding happiness and satisfaction in it will make it worth the effort.

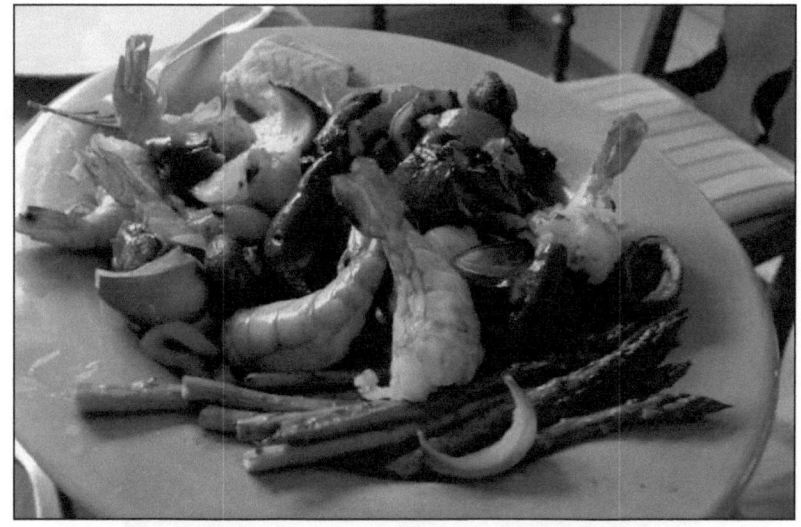

Convenient atticuse inside. I would let him first lead before you will accept some than the happing years.

CHAPTER 3

WHAT YOU NEED TO KNOW ABOUT A "RAW DIET"

Synopsis

For many years diet programs have evolved. A few of the most popular diets are the Atkins Diet, Zone Diet, Vegetarian Diet, South Beach Diet, Mediterranean Diet and Raw Food Diet. In this article we will talk about the Raw diet.

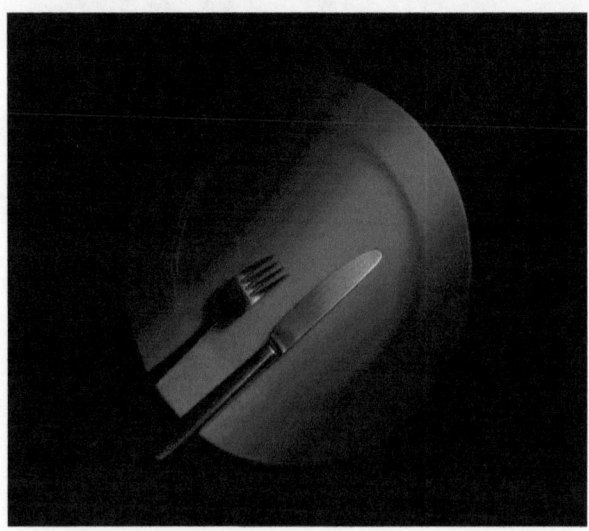

The Raw Diet

The way raw diet enthusiasts describe this regime is "it's like a magical potion handed in a salad plate". This is because its effect is delightful, it makes people feel like they don't age, and rather they grow younger. More than this, they feet that they have so much energy to do things because they feel light and teeming.

Generally, a raw diet is distinguished by food that has been heated to a certain level, normally around 104 to 115 degrees. The reason for this is that when the food is heated elaborately, the enzymes will be destroyed and when they're destroyed, we will not be able to get all the essential benefits that our body needs.

However, there are disputes to this claim and they are telling us that while it is true that cooking destroys the enzymes, eating raw food will not give much of a benefit. This is because as soon as the food reaches the acidic nature of the stomach, the enzymes will also be destroyed. Thus, the same thing occurs in whichever process you prepare the food. Having said that, the real reason why the raw diet is perceived as an effective method in maintaining a healthy weight and body is that it's a plant-based diet which is known in helping us to move in a healthier path.

Most of the raw diet enthusiasts are vegan because it is 70 to 80 percent plant-based diet. Basically, when you go for a raw diet, you should be ready to eat fresh fruits and vegetables all the time as well as other raw products such as unpasteurized milk, raw meat and the like.

On the subject of losing weight, raw diets can deliver great results as long as the rules are being followed. The general rule is to eat smaller amount of calories in order to weigh less. But the final question is, while this has several benefits, will there be a health risk that goes with the raw diet? The answer is yes! When you are practicing the raw diet, you have to avoid food poisoning as it is common when food is uncooked.

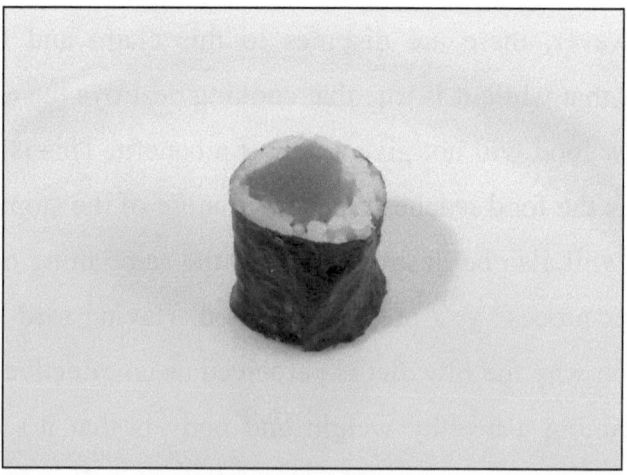

CHAPTER 4

USING JUICING FOR BETTER PHYSICAL HEALTH

Synopsis

There is no doubt that eating vegetables will make you healthy. The question is, will drinking vegetable juices give out equally healthy benefits? Or will it give more? I know you want to know the truth about juicing, that's why you are reading this. To give you this satisfaction, read on and learn more.

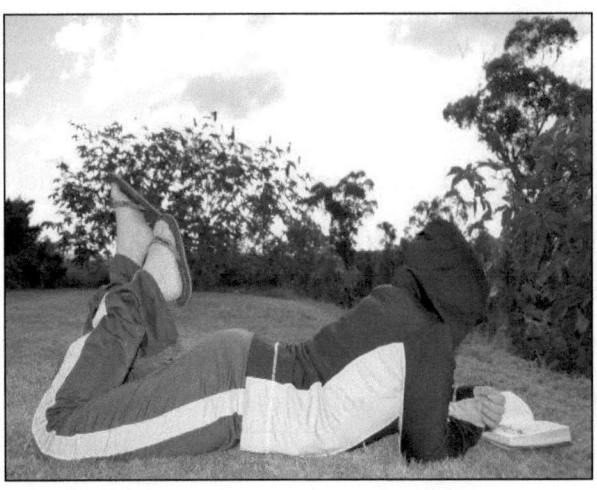

Juice It Up!

Juicing will allow you to consume more vitamins and antioxidants for an obvious reason; you can consume more vegetables when it is in liquid form compared when you eat vegetables in solid form. Studies show that drinking juice of raw vegetables help fight back chronic diseases such as immune disorders, high blood pressure, diabetes, cancers, skin diseases and many others.

Furthermore, drinking raw vegetable juices is very good for your digestion because your digestive system uses less energy to digest and liquefy food. Thus, it can rest more. Although you will not be able to benefit much on fiber, you will surely be delighted with the benefits that a live enzyme can give knowing that juicing will preserve the enzymes since the food is uncooked.

Then again, we need to understand that juices are not created the same except when done freshly. For bottled juices, make sure to read the labels because highly concentrated fruit juices can significantly increase blood sugar levels, aside from the fact that it has less nutritional value since it undergone artificial process.

To conclude, it is best to prepare fruit and vegetable juices by yourself to ensure optimum benefits. To enjoy it more, you can try combining a few types of fruits and veggies while you experiment until you find your favorites. Nevertheless, you can try some popular mixes such as blending leafy vegetable like spinach and cucumber, mixed with apple or carrot to add some sweet taste.

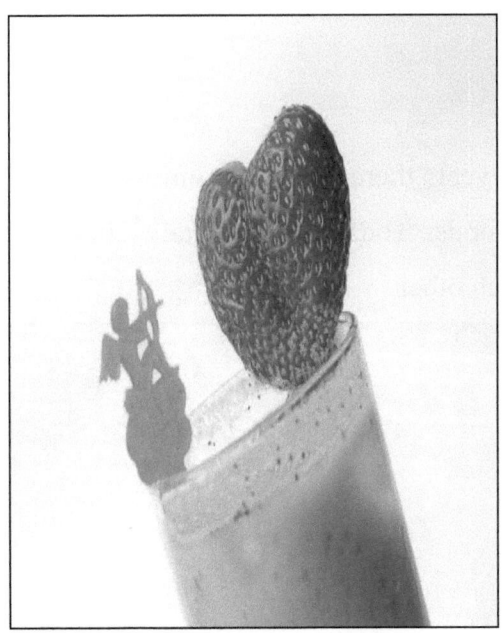

CHAPTER 5

WHAT YOU NEED TO KNOW ABOUT NATURAL AND ORGANIC FOODS

Synopsis

Over the years there has been confusion concerning natural and organic foods. Today we will talk about how these two differ from each other.

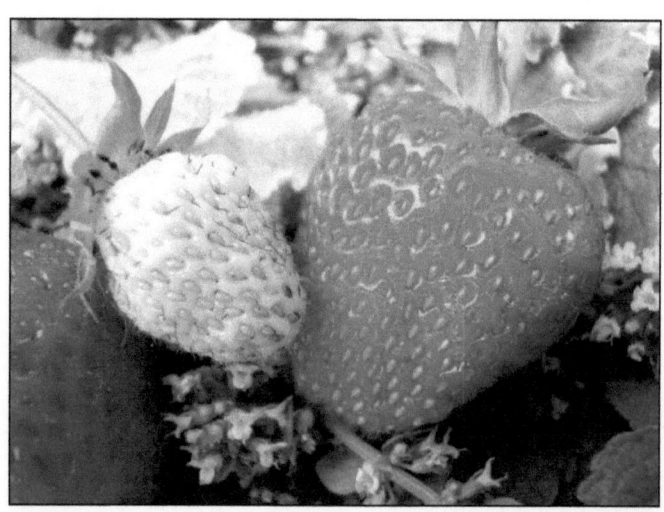

Many people cannot differentiate natural foods from organic, maybe because of how it is labeled and marketed. However, if we study deeper, there is in fact a major distinction between the two.

Know The Facts

Organic food is defined as all foods that are grown in the absence of pesticides, fertilizers, irradiation, growth hormones, antibiotics and genetic engineering. Furthermore, it is the product of organic farming where the system used in growing foods enhances biodiversity, soil biological activity and biological cycles. Natural foods on the other hand are the foods that are prepared with little or no preservatives as well as chemical additives that are usually present in other processed products.

While it is true that organic foods will lessen the chemicals and pesticides that you get from chemically processed foods, it doesn't mean that you get more health benefits out of it because even non-organic foods are still within safety levels and therefore organic foods are not necessarily more nutritious. The reason why other people choose organic foods over traditional is because it tastes better, but in terms of health, there is not much of a difference.

Furthermore, whether or not the food is organic, the chance of bacterial contamination in food is still uncontrollable. On the other hand, there are other benefits of natural and organic foods which basically include better taste as it has better firmness and texture.

CHAPTER 6

CHOOSING THE RIGHT FATS

Synopsis

We are perfectly created, therefore even fats have an important role to play. Having said this, let me describe fat first. Fat stores energy while it shields our vital organs. It is also known as the passage system of fat-soluble vitamins. Basically, we need it in our body but only in moderation. Eating fat in large amounts will make us grow heavier and will increase the chance of reaching the level of obesity.

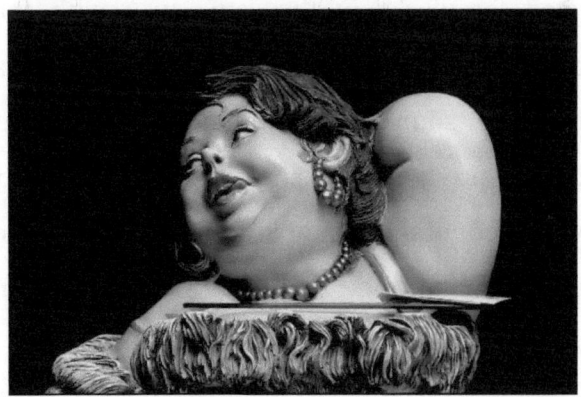

Get The Right Stuff

To stay in the health scope, we must only consume at most 55 to 60 grams of fats per day. There are several types of fat and they are categorized in two broad categories which are, "The bad fats" and "The good fats". Each type has different effects on your health.

The bad fats are identified as Trans fat and Saturated fat. When vegetable oil undergoes a certain process called hydrogenation, trans fat in formed. This process causes the oil to harden; as a result hard fats are produced. Moreover, trans fat increases bad cholesterol and decreases good cholesterol levels, this condition increases the risk of having heart disease. The most common sources of bad fats in our daily diet are fried food, cakes, pastries, cookies and the like.

Saturated fat works in the same way with trans fat. It increases bad cholesterol levels that cause heart diseases. Some of the identified sources of saturated fat are fatty meat, margarine, dairy products that contains high fat and other food prepared with coconut milk and palm-based vegetable oil.

On the other hand, the two good fats are polyunsaturated fat and monounsaturated fat. These two reduce the bad cholesterol in the body which in effect will keep the body healthy and away from chronic diseases.

Polyunsaturated fat reduces the dangers of blood clotting and decreases the risk of heart problems. Its major sources are the food rich in omega-3 like sardines, mackerel, salmon and longtail shad. Other sources are canola oil, walnuts, sunflower oil , soybean oil and the like. Monounsaturated fat also reduces bad cholesterol in the body. The foods that are rich in monounsaturated fat are peanut oils, nuts, canola oil and olive oil.

Apparently, it is easier to exceed fats consumption than to stay in average. But now that you already know the types of fats and their benefits, always choose the good over the bad. Also, strive to consume fats in moderation as even good fats when taken excessively can be harmful to your health.

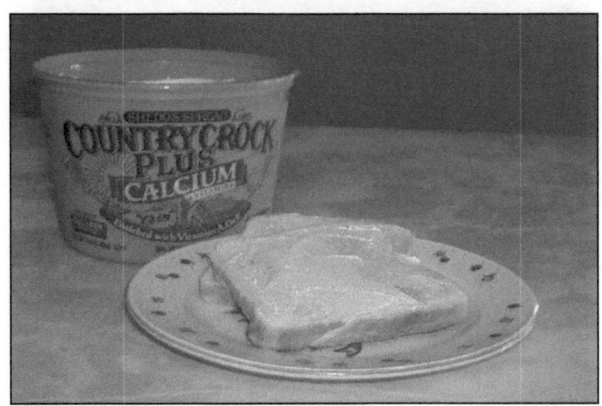

CHAPTER 7

CHOOSING THE CARBS

Synopsis

Dietary carbohydrates, also known as saccharine have actual sugars and starches that are responsible in providing energy to humans, animals and even plants. Carbs in a real sense have advantages and disadvantages, especially since right now food production has dramatically changed as well as how food is consumed.

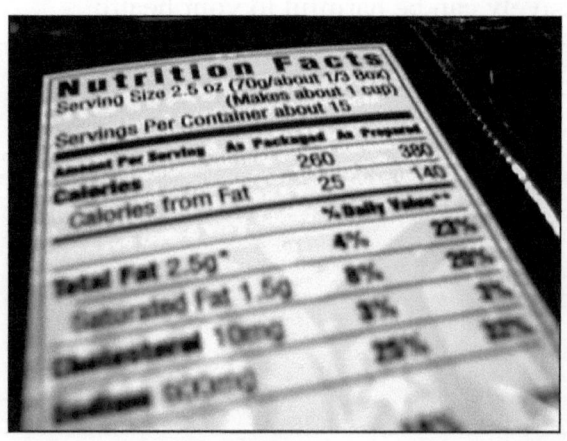

Proper Selection

Carbs have two types, monosaccharides and polysaccharides. Monosaccharides can be easily digested and absorbed by the body. It is normally obtained in fruits and specific dairy products. Other sources of simple carbohydrates are pastas, white bread and white sugar.

Polysaccharides on the other hand take a longer period of time to be digested and absorbed by the body. It is normally found in vegetables, legumes, whole grain breads, brown rice and the like. Basically, unrefined grains are a good sources of complex carbs compared to refined grains, this is because the filtering process generally removes the fiber and nutrients present in grains. Therefore, eating unrefined grain products will give you lasting energy.

While carbs are essential in the body, we must make sure that we are picking the right carbs to consume. To do that, we need to understand carbs even better and know how to use them in our advantage. The catch is, we need to eat the right carbs that our body needs in order for us to sustain the right energy.

It is recommended by the experts that for an adult's dietary energy, 40 to 65% percent of it must come from carbs and around 10% of it should be simple carbs. Too many cravings of high-glycemic foods will not only make us fat but also increases the risk of acquiring diabetes.

Talking about diabetes and weight problems, cutting all carbs in your diet is definitely not the solution. Carbohydrates are very important in providing our body with enough nutrients, vitamins and soluble fiber that is good in maintaining healthy sugar and cholesterol levels.

So how do we choose the right carbs? Here's how. Switch from low- glycemic foods and reduce calorie intake to at most 250-500 calories per day. Moreover, allow yourself to consume 20g to 35g of fiber in a day. One of the best sources of fiber is whole grain foods.

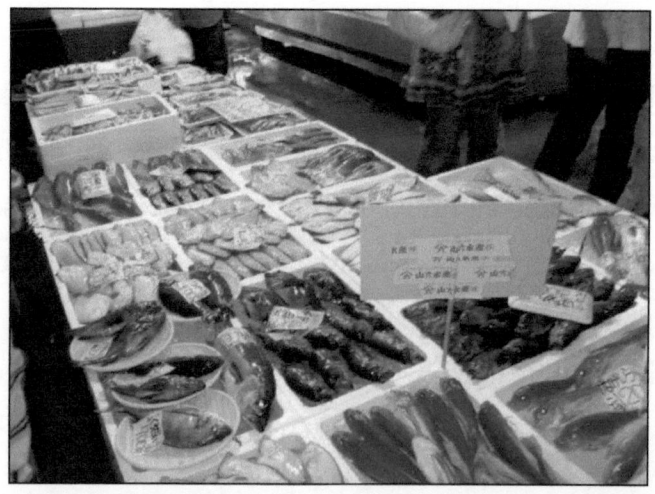

Protein is known as very low in carbs. Consume foods that are lean in protein such as notfat dairy products, skinless poultry, tofu, legumes and fish. On the other hand, you must avoid foods that are high in saturated fats like pork, high-fat dairy products and beef.

CHAPTER 8

WHAT DOES IT MEAN TO YOUR HEALTH
TO BE A VEGETARIAN

Synopsis

A vegetarian is a person who prefers eating vegetables and no meat at all. However, it does not mean that they don't eat foods other than vegetables, they still eat other food but strictly no meat. Many people try to go vegetarian because of health and weight loss benefits. Studies show that cutting some meat into your diet will give you more benefits in terms of achieving healthy weight and body.

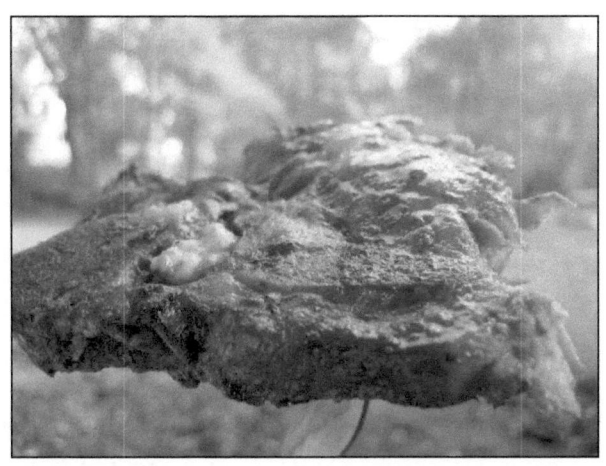

Know The Facts

A lot of people are lured to vegetarianism for many different reasons. Some want to live healthier and longer, others would love to preserve animals and there are some who just want to shed some pounds through eating pure vegetables.

There is something you need to understand about being a vegetarian. Vegetarian diets will protect you against most types of diseases, including heart disease and cancer. In the U.S., around 1 million people died because of cardiovascular diseases and right now it is considered as one of the major causes of mortality in the U.S.

In addition, vegetarian diet patrons acquire more fiber than those of meat eaters. This is because veggies are rich in fiber and at the same time they are high in antioxidants that will keep you healthy and younger looking.

Being vegetarian is also effective in losing weight because it is plant based. What is good about it is that you lose weight without even measuring the calories that you have consumed and best of all you don't feel hungry as you can eat whenever you want to. The more vegetables you eat the more fiber you get that can help you regulate your bowels which is also a good prevention for colon cancer.

More than achieving a healthy weight is attaining a healthy body and a longer life. Research shows that when you switch to a healthier vegetarian diet, you are adding 13 more years to your existence. This is especially true when you go for a low calorie diet, unrefined complex carbs, and soy and fiber-rich foods.

Vegetarians also enjoy high amounts of calcium from calcium-rich vegetables like broccoli, collards, kale and turnip greens. Other great sources of calcium that are present in vegetarian diets is soymilk, dry beans and tofu.

Ultimately, aside from having strong bones, you will also experience more energy that you need to last the day. It provides longer vigor since eating vegetables will prevent your bloodstream from clotting, giving a good passage way for oxygen to be used by the body. Therefore, a vegetarian diet will keep you energetic all throughout the day.

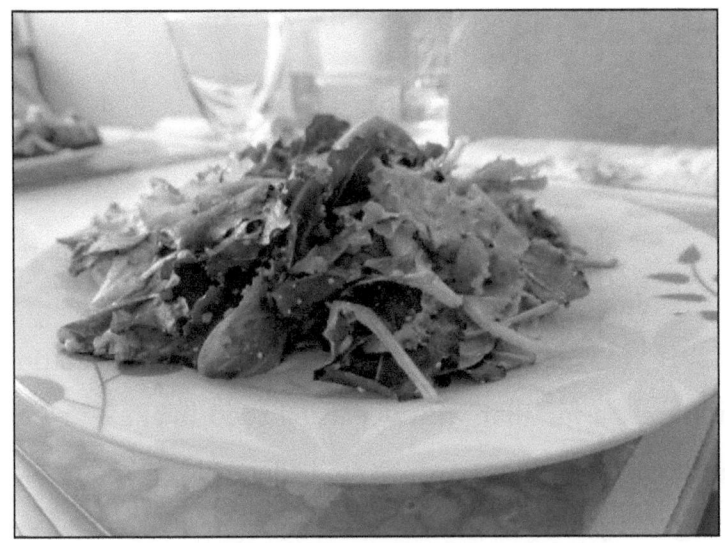

CHAPTER 9

FOODS TO KICK TO THE CURB

Synopsis

I know most of us can relate when I say that there will always be that bad food that we don't want to give up no matter how badly we want to get healthy and fit. What we can do is to identify and be familiar with our usual food intake. We can list down all of those foods we eat and identify the foods that we need to give up or consume in strict moderation.

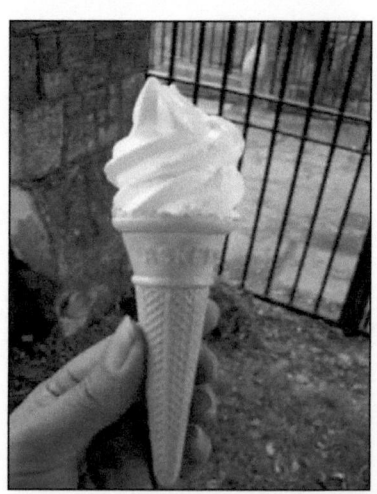

What To Avoid

To guide us through this, we can consider the below guidelines to help us succeed in keeping our body fit. Generally, we should know as to what level we should be avoiding such foods.

First in the list is red meat. If we want to stay healthy we need to throw out red meat from our diet as it will not give us any good. It is best that we go for white meat instead. Next would be frozen and processed food. These foods are high in calories and contain preservative chemicals. The majority of us are consuming frozen and processed foods because of the convenience it brings. However, we must pay greater attention to our health than our convenience.

Also, we are well aware that fast foods are not good at all. Kick it out to give way to healthier and tastier foods. Soft drinks are one big temptation. A lot of people are addicted to sodas. If you are one of them now is a high time for you to give up your favorite soda and let your body become chemical and sugar free. When you do that, your body will thank you forever.

Alcoholic drinks are definitely included in the list. It is not bad to drink alcohol when taken in moderation. However, if you want to lose weight while obtaining a healthy body, it is best to just drop the idea of drinking. Normally we can avoid drinking alcohol if we have illnesses that we need to treat, therefore pulling out from alcoholic drinks is definitely possible.

Lastly, when all the aforementioned foods are eliminated in your regime, you can be sure that you will become healthier and leaner. Of course it will not happen in an instant and things will happen gradually. Don't leave off and continue changing for the better, one day you will wake up and you will be used to it. You will realize that keeping yourself healthy is not a challenge anymore, but a regular part of your system.

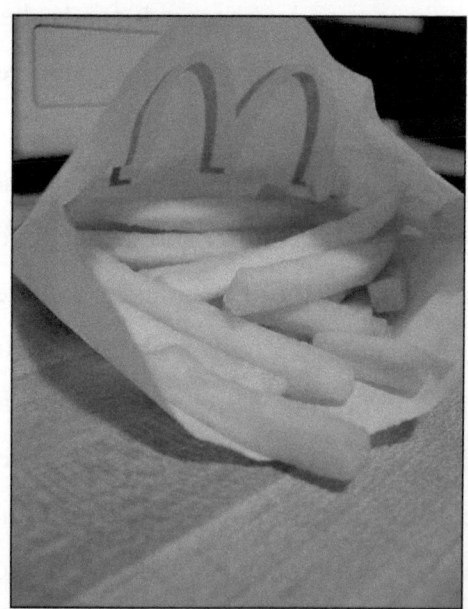

CHAPTER 10

THE BENEFITS OF EATING RIGHT
FOR A HEALTHY BODY

Synopsis

As we are all know, eating the right foods in the right amounts will give us the maximum benefits. However, most of us are not well educated on the right types of food that are needed by our body to function properly. Some of us don't even know when to just stop eating. When we eat the right kind of food we are allowing the body to be properly nourished. Hence, as a result we will be able to gain health benefits from our healthful efforts.

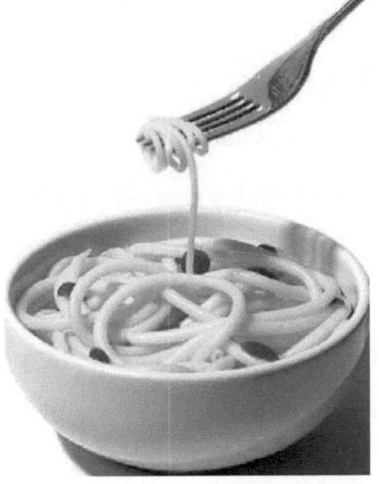

The Rewards

There are several benefits of eating the right food. Below is the list.

1. Maintains a healthy body weight
2. Maintains a normal blood sugar level
3. Reduces the risk of heart attacks
4. Reduces the risk of cancer
5. Improves good blood circulation and maintains stable energy levels

However, despite the above mentioned benefits a lot of people still tend to avoid eating right for the reason that they are under the impression that whether or not they eat good food, there is not much of a difference in their health status. Others tend to evade eating the right food because they cannot afford to live in such a healthy lifestyle.

It is true that each of us have different needs. Thus, it would be better if we discover and explore more healthful ideas that will best suit us. In general, health professionals always recommend eating the right food for a healthier body.

A healthy diet is composed of protein, fats, carbohydrates, vitamins, minerals and water. These elements need to be taken in proportion to be able to get optimum results.

The good thing about this idea, when you start eating the right foods, there is a possibility that your family and friends will begin to follow. Aside from that, when you start a good habit and strive to really carry on with it, chances are you will become more motivated to continue what you are doing. Thus, staying away from unhealthy foods will never be that difficult again.

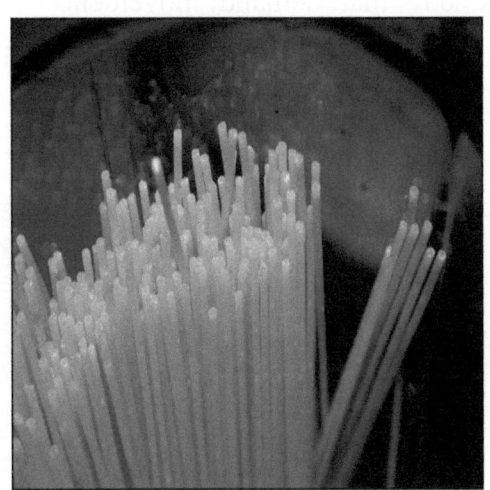

CHAPTER 11

EXERCISE BASICS

Physical activity is specified as movement that demands contraction of your muscles. Any of the actions we do throughout the day that demand movement - housekeeping, gardening, walking, climbing up stairs - are illustrations of physical activity.

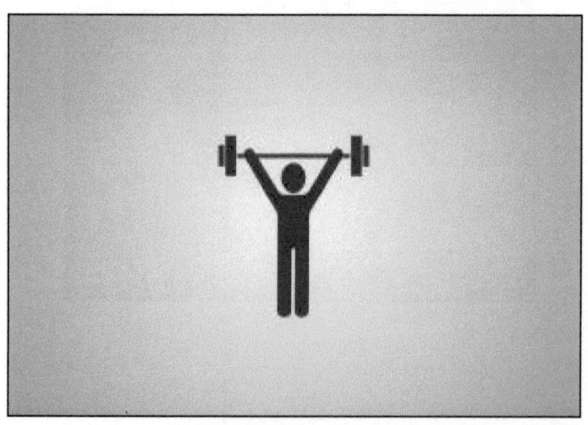

The Basics

Exercise is a particular form of physical activity - planned, purposeful physical activity executed with the intent of gaining fitness or other health advantages. Exercising at a health club, swimming, cycling, running, and sports, like golf and tennis, are all kinds of exercise.

How can you tell if an action is considered moderate or vigorous in intensity level? If you are able to talk although executing it, it's moderate. If you have to stop to catch your breath after saying simply a couple of words, it's vigorous.

Depending upon your fitness level, a game of doubles tennis would likely be moderate in intensity level, although a singles game could be more vigorous. Also, ballroom dance would be moderate, however aerobic dance could be considered vigorous. Once again, it's not simply your choice of activity, its how much effort it demands.

Ideally, an exercise regimen should include elements designed to better each of these components:

Cardio-respiratory endurance. Better your respiratory endurance - your ability to engage in aerobics - through actions like brisk walking, jogging, running, cycling, swimming, jumping rope, rowing, or cross-country skiing. As you reach distance or intensity level goals, reset them higher or shift to a different action to keep challenging yourself.

Muscular force. You are able to better muscular strength most efficiently by lifting weights, utilizing either free weights like barbells and dumbbells or lifting machines.

Muscular endurance. Better your endurance with calisthenics (conditioning exercises), weight training, and actions like running or swimming.

Flexibleness. Work to better your level of flexibility through stretching exercises that are done as part of your exercise or through a discipline like yoga or pilates that contains stretching.

Although it's possible to handle all of these fitness factors with a physically active life-style, an exercise program should help you accomplish even greater advantages.

Increasing the sum of physical activity in your daily life is a great beginning - like parking a couple of blocks from your destination to get in a little walking. However to truly accomplish fitness goals, you'll need to incorporate structured, vigorous actions into your schedule to help you accomplish even more of your fitness and health goals.

CHAPTER 12

SET YOUR GOAL AND STICK TO IT

Starting or getting back to a workout routine involves more than simply scheduling your exercises and joining a gym. As a matter of fact, it's totally possible to join a gym and never really go, even as those monthly payments appear on your bank statement. I understand this because I've done that a couple of times in my life. Sticking to your goals demands a couple of mental tricks to help keep you going, centered and motivated.

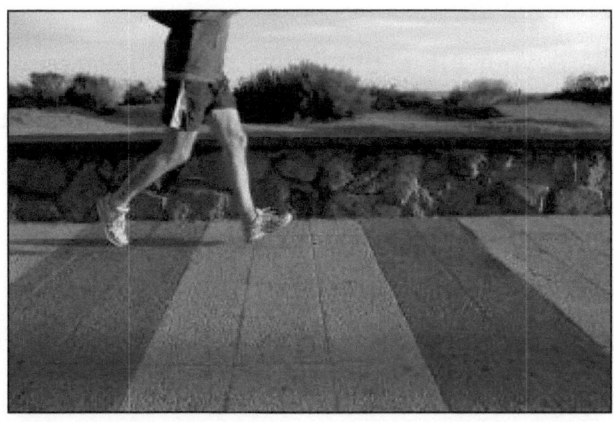

Keep Going

Momentum is a central part of uniform exercise. It's normal to have those weeks when everything goes correctly: You do all your exercises, eat like a health nut and begin to think, 'I may completely accomplish this!'

Then 'it' materializes. 'It' may be a vacation, an illness...something that throws you off your game. Getting back is constantly tough, partly as you've lost that momentum. We already realize that an object at rest tends to remain at rest, so getting going again is the only way to get your momentum moving.

Rather than caring about making up for lost time with intense exercises, center on simply getting some exercise time in. Plan your exercises for the week and call yourself successful simply for turning up.

Purchase yourself a little something like a new pair of running shoes or an exceptional pair of shorts to wear to the gym. If you're having hassles getting back to it, get a new outfit or download a few new songs to your MP3 player so you've something to look forward to.

Make an appointment to exercise with an acquaintance or call your gym and arrange a free consultation with a personal trainer. Even if you don't sign on, getting back into the exercise environment may be just what you need.

If the thought of coming back to boring gym exercises makes you want to die, do something completely different. Sign on for a local belly dance class or check into that new yoga studio. A switch of scenery and a brand new activity may refresh and rejuvenate you.

Picture this: you're at a party and you've promised yourself you won't scarf down the buffet like a famished maniac. Then you see a huge platter of the prettiest cheese you've ever came across. Many hours later, feeling your cheese hangover start, you vow to make up for it tomorrow with a long workout.

There are some issues with this approach - first, you can't undo what you consumed the night before and, secondly, killing yourself with an exercise isn't a good answer as it makes you hate exercise even more.

If you're busy living in yesterday's errors, many of your decisions will be founded on guilt and shame instead of what you really want (and need) to accomplish to achieve your goals. Real change comes from day-to-day choices and becoming mindful and basing your choices on what you need now (rather than what you did or didn't do yesterday) will make your exercise life much more passable.

CHAPTER 13

GET YOUR EXERCISE PLAN TOGETHER

Taking the time to really sit down and make a concrete schedule is the essential first step towards building the body you want. Following comes the tough task of following it each week, but that's a different topic for a different day, for now let's just center on putting a workout schedule together.

Putting A Plan Together

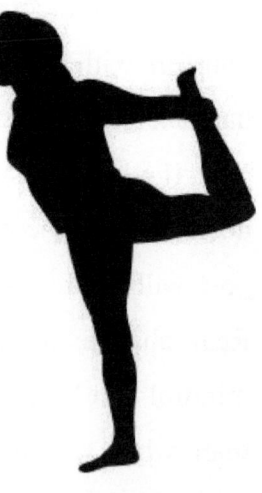

1. Sit with a weekly calendar and ascertain how many days of the week you're willing to workout.

2. Choose what particular sort of workout you wish to engage in. For example, cardiovascular workout will help

you lose fat, whereas lifting weights will form muscle.

3. Devote yourself to exercising according to your plan. This is the most crucial step.

4. Abide by your schedule for at the least one month. The gains you'll see after 4 weeks ought to be decent to keep you motivated.

Cardiovascular workout

1. Integrate 30-minute workout sessions into your schedule. 30 minutes of every day workouts is enough for most individuals.

2. Decide on a sort of cardiovascular workout for a particular day of the week. Utilizing a treadmill or stair-climbing machine, jogging, bicycling, and swimming are all efficient forms of cardiovascular workout.

3. Warm up and actively stretch out for five minutes prior to starting any activity.

4. Workout at a moderate pace for twenty minutes.

5. Follow up with a five minute cool down.

6. Switch your schedule to fit longer workout periods if suitable.

7. Stick with your schedule.

Weights

1. Allow thirty to sixty minute workout sessions for weights. If you don't spend much time socializing or resting during your workout you are able to get a great session of lifting done in that time. Do not rest more than sixty seconds between sets.

2. Start by doing total body workouts aimed at conditioning each major muscle group (upper body, lower body and back). Equilibrated development is exceedingly crucial.

3. Divide your workouts as you get to be a more experienced lifter. This will enable you to better center on particular muscle groups and areas. A basic split that targets each major muscle group is: chest and triceps, back and biceps, shoulder and legs.

4. Rest your muscles in between sessions. Allow each muscle group to rest at least one day between sessions. Your muscles can not grow unless they have time to rest and mend.

5. Tailor your agenda to best fulfill your goals.

6. Stick with your workout schedule.

CHAPTER 14

MAKE SURE TO WARM UP

Many athletes perform some sort of regular warm-up and cool off during training and racing.

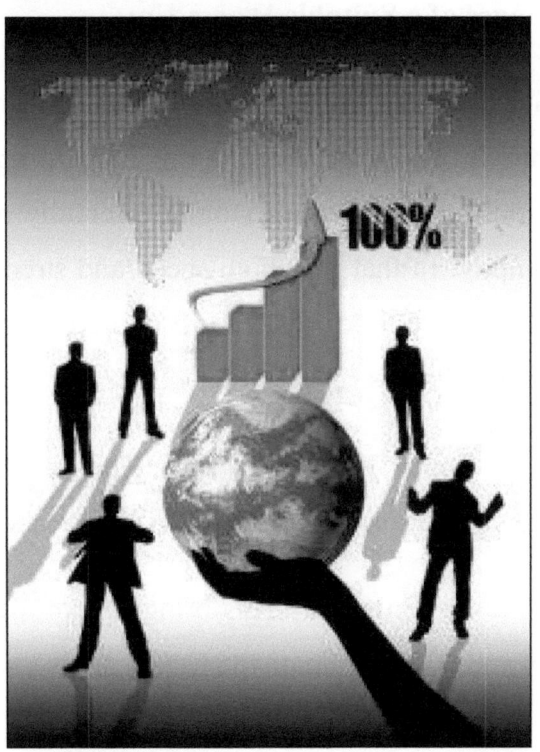

A suitable warm up may step-up the blood flow to the working muscle which results in diminished muscle stiffness, less risk of trauma and bettered performance. Additional advantages of warming up include physiologic and psychological preparation.

Warm Up

Advantages of a Suitable Warm Up:

Modified Muscle Temperature - The temperature step-ups inside muscles that are utilized during a warm-up routine. A warmed up muscle both contracts more forcefully and loosens up more promptly. In that way both speed and strength may be heightened. Likewise, the chance of pulling a muscle and causing trauma is far less.

Modified Body Temperature - This betters muscle elasticity, likewise cutting back the risk of strains and pulls.

Blood Vessels Enlarge - This brings down the resistance to blood flow and lower strain on the heart.

Better Efficient Cooling - By triggering the heat-dissipation mechanisms in the body (effective sweating) an athlete may cool expeditiously and help preclude overheating early in the event or race.

Modified Blood Temperature - The temperature of blood increases as it goes through the muscles. As blood temperature climbs, the binding of oxygen to hemoglobin de-escalates so oxygen is more readily useable for working muscles, which might better endurance.

Bettered Range of Motion - The range of motion around a joint is modified.

Hormonal Shifts - Your body step-ups its production of assorted hormones responsible for regulating energy production. During warm-up this equilibrium of hormones makes more carbs and fatty acids available for energy manufacturing.

Mental Prep - The warm-up is likewise a great time to mentally prepare for an event by clearing the mind, increasing centering, critiquing skills and technique. Favorable imagery may likewise relax the athlete and establish concentration.

Typical Warm up exercises include:

Bit by bit increasing the intensity of your particular sport. This utilizes the particular skills of a sport and is occasionally called a related warm-up. For runners, the idea is to jog for a while and add a few sprints into the routine to engage all the muscle fibers.

Adding motions not related to your sport in a slow steadfast fashion: calisthenics or flexibility exercises for instance. Ball players frequently utilize unrelated workout for their warm up.

Which to pick? The best time to stretch a muscle is after it has a modified blood flow and has modified temperature to prevent trauma. Stretching out a cold muscle may increase the risk of trauma from pulls and tears.

So you're better off doing gradual aerobic workout prior to stretching. Bear in mind that the best time to stretch is after your workout as your muscles are warm and pliable with the increase of blood in them. Make certain your warm up starts out gradually, and utilizes the muscles that will be strained during workout.

Keep in mind that the perfect warm up is a very individual process that may only come with practice, experimentation and experience. Try warming up in various ways, at various intensities until you find what works best for you.

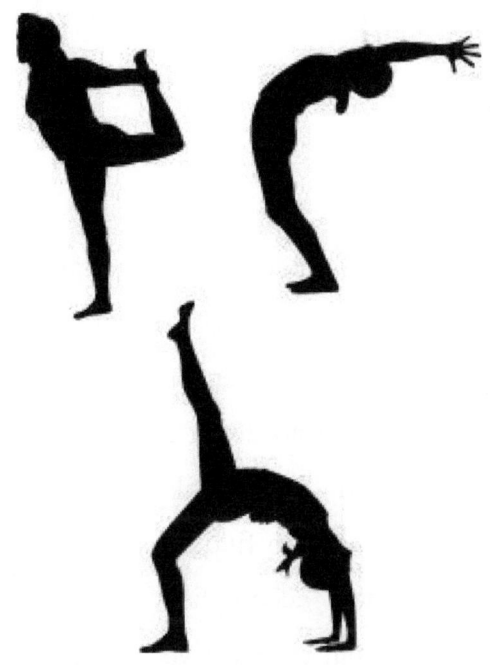

CHAPTER 15

INCORPORATE CARDIO TRAINING

With a big share of Americans overweight, it's clear that a lot of us are not abiding by the most recent exercise guidelines dictating up to an hour of exercise every day. In fact, there is no doubt a collective groan when individuals recognized they'd now have to find an hour every day to accomplish something they can't seem to find five minutes for. How crucial are these guidelines and what may you do to make them fit into your life?

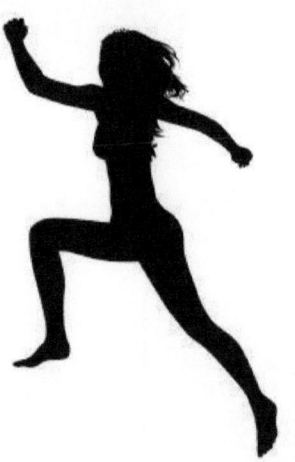

Cardio Basics

Before we get started, you ought to at least know why it's so crucial. Cardiovascular exercise merely means that you're involved in an activity that elevates your heart rate to a level where you're working, but may still talk (also known as, in your Target Heart Rate). Here's why cardio is so crucial:

- It's one way to burn off calories and help you slim down

- It makes your heart strong so that it doesn't have to work as grueling to pump blood

- It step-ups your lung capacity

- It helps bring down risk of heart attack, elevated cholesterol, hypertension and diabetes

- It makes you feel great

- It aids you in sleeping better

- It helps bring down tension

- I could go on all day, however you get the point

Bottom line: you require cardio if you want to get your weight in check and get your tension to a tolerable level.

The opening move is to what kind of activities you'd like to do. The trick is to consider what's accessible to you, what fits your personality and what you'd feel comfy fitting into your life.

If you like to go outside, running, bicycling, hiking or walking are all great choices. If you love the gym, you'll have access to stationary bicycles, elliptical trainers, treadmills, row machines, stair masters and more.

For the home exerciser, there are a number of first-class workout videos to try and you don't require much equipment to get an exceptional home cardio workout.

Bear in mind, you might not know what sort of activity you enjoy yet. That's all part of the experience, so don't be frightened to try something and, if it doesn't work, go on to something else.

Just about any activity will work, provided it demands a motion that gets your heart rate into your Target Zone. Remember:

There's no 'most proficient' cardio exercise. Anything that you like and that gets your heart rate up fills the bill

It's not what you do, but how hard you work. Any exercise may be challenging if you make it that way

Do something you love. If you detest gym workouts, don't force yourself onto a treadmill. If you love socializing, think about sports, group fitness, exercising with an acquaintance or a walking club.

Pick out something you can see yourself doing at least three days a week.

Be flexible and don't be frightened to branch out once you get well- situated with exercise.

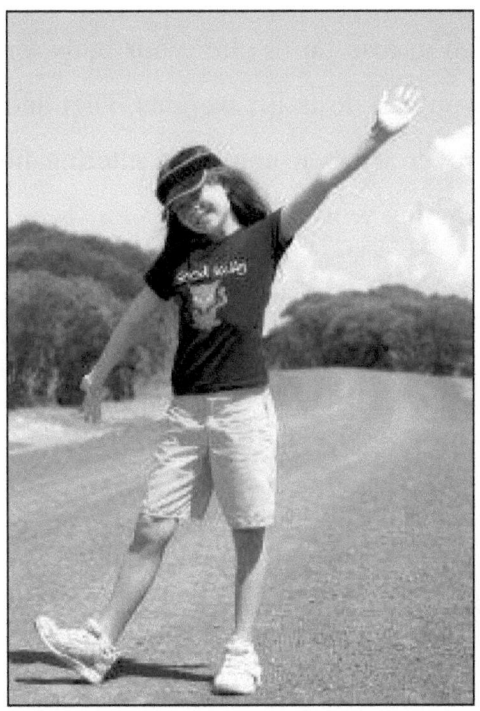

CHAPTER 16

USE WEIGHTS

If you wish to lose fat or alter your body, one of the most crucial things you can do is lift weights. Diet and cardio are as important, however when it comes to altering how your body looks, weight training wins handily.

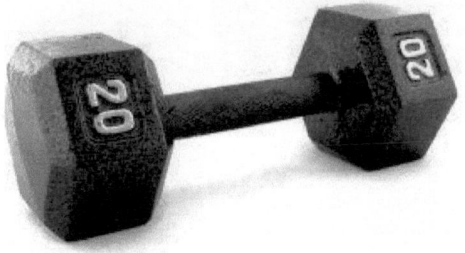

Lifting Basics

If you've hesitated to begin a strength training regimen, it might motivate you to know that lifting weights can:

Help elevate your metabolism. Muscle burns off a lot of calories t, so the more muscle you have, the more calories you'll burn off all day long.

- Fortify bones, particularly crucial for women
- Make you stronger and better muscular endurance
- Help you prevent injuries
- Better your confidence and self-pride
- Better coordination and balance

Getting going with strength training may be confusing - what exercises can you do? How many sets and reps? How much lifting? The routine you pick out will be based on your fitness goals as well as the tools you have available and the time you have for exercises.

If you're establishing your own program, you'll have to understand some basic strength training rules. These rules will teach you how to make certain you're utilizing adequate weight, determine your sets and reps and insure you're always advancing in your workouts.

To build muscle, you have to utilize more resistance than your muscles are used to. This is crucial as the more you do, the more your body is capable of doing, so you ought to increase your workload to prevent plateaus. In plain language, this implies you ought to be lifting enough weight that you may just complete the desired number of reps. You ought to be able to finish your last rep with difficulty but likewise with great form.

To prevent plateaus (or adaptation), you have to increase your intensity regularly. You are able to do this by increasing the amount of weight lifted, altering your sets/reps, altering the exercises and altering the sort of resistance. You are able to make these alterations on a weekly or monthly basis.

Specificity. This principle means you ought to train for your goal. That means, if you wish to increase your strength, your regimen ought to be designed around that goal (e.g., train with bigger weights closer to your 1 RM (1 rep max)). To slim down, select an assortment of rep ranges to target assorted muscle fibers.

Rest days are even as crucial as workout days. It's during these respites that your muscles grow and change, so make certain you're not working the same muscle groups 2 days in a row.

Before you get going on setting up your routine, keep a couple of key points in mind:

Constantly warm up before you begin lifting weights. This helps get your muscles warm and prevent trauma. You may warm up with light cardio or by doing a light set of every exercise before moving to heavier weights.

Elevate and lower your weights slowly. Don't utilize momentum to lift the weight. If you have to swing to get the weight up, probabilities are you're utilizing too much weight.

Don't hold your breath and make certain you're utilizing full range of motion throughout the motion.

Stand up straight. Pay attention to your posture and use your abs in every motion you're doing to keep your balance and protect your spine.

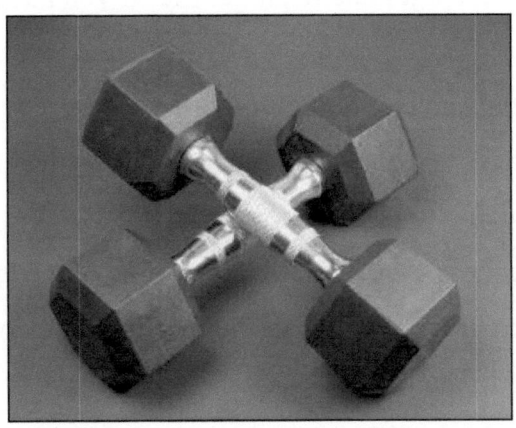

CHAPTER 17

THE BENEFITS TO A HEALTHY LIFESTYLE OTHER THAN LOOKING GREAT

The first advantage of living a healthy life-style is that you likely will live a longer and healthier life. If you have a family to support this is really important as you'll be there for them to supply financial and emotional support.

If you have a son or daughter I'm sure that they'll want their mom and dad to be there for them.

For parents you get the joy of raising your youngsters and watching them grow from tot to their early childhood years and all the way up to maturity.

As a parent you'll have the joy of being around your grand kids and even watch them grow.

Advantages

A different advantage of a healthy life-style is that you'll be more vibrant and have more energy. You'll have more get up and go. This will let you be more active and achieve more. This will allow you to have a more favorable attitude in life and will help out your physical, emotional and mental frame of mind.

It will let you be more productive at home and at work. You will not have as many sick days at work therefore making you a more generative employee. If you have a business, this expanded productivity may help your company be more fruitful. Overall this expanded productivity may result in great financial dividends for you in the future.

Overall you'll look and feel better. You'll have a much more positive outlook on life. It will pay dandy dividends for you down the road as far as your physical, emotional and mental frame of mind. It will bring down tension and stress. It likewise will ease and decrease the chances of depressive disorder or getting depressed all the time as you are feeling great about yourself and have a more positive frame of mind.

It's a form of preventive health care and preventative medicine. It will help prevent heart conditions, cancer and many additional debilitating diseases.

I'm saving the best for last. Among the greatest advantages of living a healthy lifestyle is the amount of cash you'll save. When you're healthy you'll;

- Spend less time and cash on physician visits
- Spend less cash on prescriptions
- Fewer if any visits to the hospital
- Lessen the risks of out of control medical expenses

which is among the leading causes of bankruptcy and financial destruction.

Regrettably, very few individuals recognize and understand the advantages that a healthy life-style may have on ones bank account.

So these are the advantages of healthy lifestyle and overall how to live a healthy life-style.

Wrapping Up

Maintaining a healthy body and mind really is not that difficult of a task. In reality, part of the hardest part is making the decision to make some changes in your lifestyle. The sooner you can be honest with yourself about the choices you make in your life the sooner you can begin to live healthy. Properly maintaining your body is key to handling the stresses of everyday life. It is also crucial in maintaining energy levels we need to accomplish our daily tasks. Take the first step in changing your health by utilizing the steps and tips from the above book. Bear in mind that there's more to a beautiful body than just utilizing effective wellness products. You need to be on a total preventative healthcare and wellness program that involves diet, nutrition (making a point that your body gets the proper nutrients) and exercise. All it takes is practice and effort, good luck!

Printed by Libri Plureos GmbH in Hamburg, Germany